NUTRIENT-RICH DIET FOR IMMUNITY

Ultimate Guide To Boosting The Immune System

ALLISON REESE

TABLE OF CONTENTS

INTRODUCTION

In the ever-changing health and wellness landscape, bolstering your immune system is a cornerstone for a resilient and thriving life. The immune system, a complex network of cells, tissues, and organs, serves as the body's defence against invaders. From combating common colds to thwarting more serious threats, a robust immune system plays a pivotal role in maintaining overall well-being. This guide delves into the strategies and practices aimed at boosting your immunity. We'll explore the intricate workings of the immune system, uncover the impact of nutrition, sleep, and exercise, and provide practical insights into fostering a strong defence against illness. Whether you're navigating the challenges of a fast-paced lifestyle or seeking proactive measures for long-term health, the journey to fortify your immune resilience begins here. Join us as we unravel the science behind immune support and embark on a path toward a healthier, more resilient you.

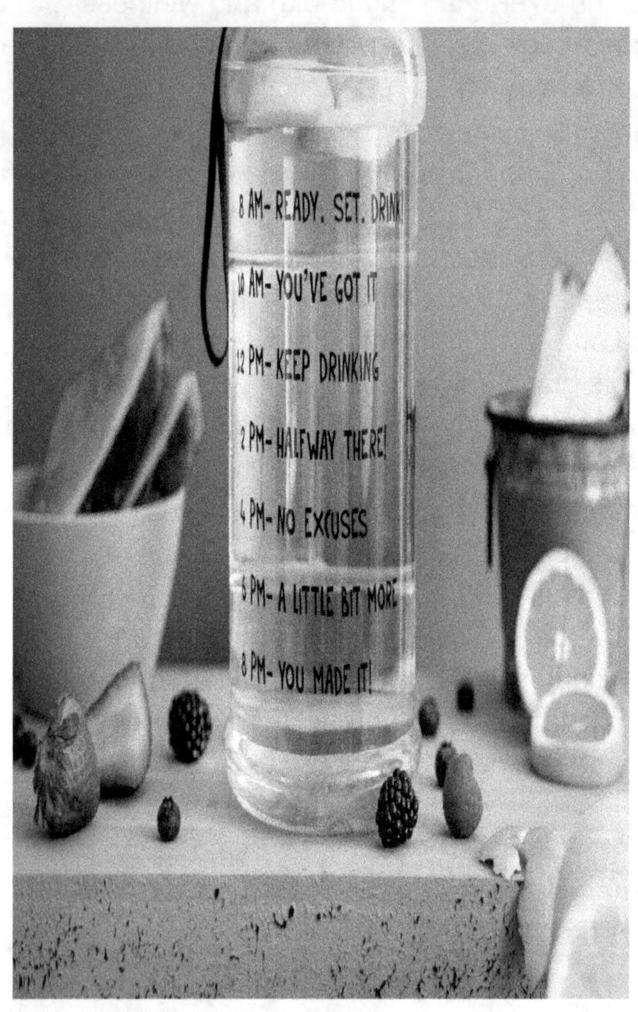

8 AM- READY. SET. DRINK!
10 AM- YOU'VE GOT IT
12 PM- KEEP DRINKING
2 PM- HALFWAY THERE!
4 PM- NO EXCUSES
6 PM- A LITTLE BIT MORE
8 PM- YOU MADE IT!

CHAPTER ONE

UNDERSTANDING THE IMMUNE SYSTEM

The immune system is a complex and intricate network of cells, tissues, and organs that work together to defend the body against harmful invaders, such as bacteria, viruses, fungi, and other pathogens. Its primary function is to recognize and eliminate these foreign substances while distinguishing them from the body's healthy cells. A well-functioning immune system is crucial for maintaining overall health and preventing infections and diseases.

Key Components of the Immune System:

- ❖ **White Blood Cells (Leukocytes):**
    - ➢ The immune system's main cellular constituents are white blood cells.
    - ➢ There are different types of white blood cells, including neutrophils, lymphocytes, monocytes, eosinophils, and basophils, each

with specific functions in the
immune response.

❖ **Lymphatic System:**
  ➢ The lymphatic system is a
    network of vessels, nodes, and
    organs that transport lymph, a
    fluid containing white blood cells,
    throughout the body.
  ➢ Lymph nodes act as filters,
    trapping and destroying
    pathogens as lymph passes
    through.

❖ **Bone Marrow:**
  ➢ White blood cells, among other
    blood cells, are produced in the
    bone marrow.
  ➢ Stem cells in the bone marrow
    differentiate into various types of
    blood cells, contributing to the
    continuous renewal of the
    immune system.

- ❖ **Thymus:**
    - ➢ The thymus is a gland located in the chest that plays a crucial role in the development and maturation of T lymphocytes (T cells), a type of white blood cell.
    - ➢ T cells are essential for cell-mediated immunity and help coordinate the immune response.

- ❖ **Spleen:**
    - ➢ The spleen acts as a blood filter and immune organ.
    - ➢ It helps remove damaged blood cells and serves as a reservoir for immune cells.

- ❖ **Antibodies:**
    - ➢ Antibodies, also known as immunoglobulins, are proteins produced by B lymphocytes (B cells).
    - ➢ Antibodies recognize and bind to specific pathogens, marking them

for destruction by other immune cells.

- ❖ **Complement System:**
  - ➤ The complement system consists of proteins that enhance the ability of antibodies and phagocytic cells to clear microbes and damaged cells from an organism.

How the Immune System Works:

Recognition:

The immune system recognizes foreign invaders by detecting specific molecules on their surface, known as antigens.

- ❖ **Activation:**
  - ➤ Upon recognition, immune cells are activated to mount a response. This involves the production of antibodies, mobilization of white blood cells,

and coordination of various
immune components.

❖ **Attack and Elimination:**
  ➢ The immune system deploys
    white blood cells to attack and
    eliminate the invaders. This may
    involve phagocytosis (engulfing
    and digesting pathogens), the
    release of toxic substances, and
    the activation of specialized
    immune cells.

❖ **Memory:**
  ➢ After an infection is cleared, the
    immune system retains a
    memory of the encountered
    pathogen. This memory allows
    for a faster and more effective
    response upon subsequent
    exposure to the same pathogen,
    providing immunity.

Factors Influencing Immune Function:

The immune system's efficacy can be influenced by several things, such as:

- **Nutrition:** A well-balanced diet with essential nutrients supports immune function.
- **Sleep:** Adequate and quality sleep is crucial for a healthy immune system.
- **Exercise:** Regular physical activity contributes to overall health and enhances immune function.
- **Stress:** Stress: An immune system that is under constant stress can become compromised.
- **Vaccination:** Immunization helps the immune system recognize and remember specific pathogens, protecting against infections.

→ In summary, the immune system is a dynamic defence mechanism that plays a vital role in maintaining health. Understanding its components, functions, and the factors that influence

its efficacy is essential for promoting
overall well-being and preventing illness.

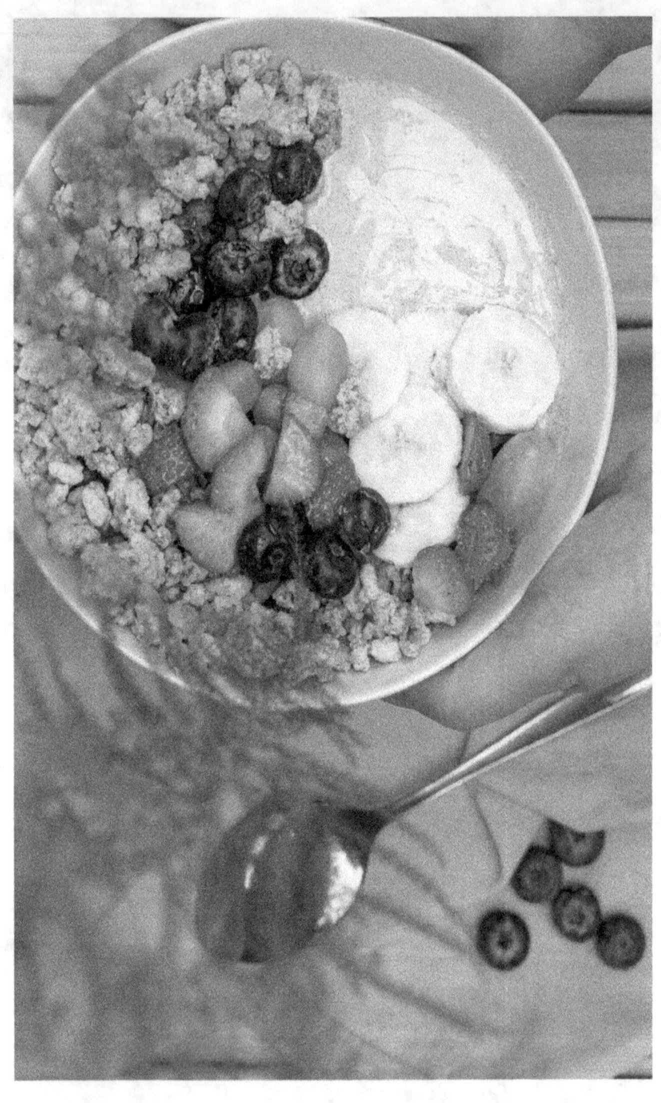

CHAPTER TWO

NUTRIENT-RICH DIET FOR THE IMMUNE SYSTEM

Maintaining a nutrient-rich diet is crucial for supporting a robust immune system, providing the body with the essential elements to fend off infections and promote overall well-being. Here's a breakdown of key nutrients and the foods that are rich sources:

- ❖ **Vitamins and Minerals:**
  - ➢ **Vitamin C:** Citrus fruits (oranges and lemons), strawberries, bell peppers, and broccoli are high in vitamin C.
  - ➢ **Vitamin D:** Abundant in fatty fish (salmon, mackerel), fortified dairy products, and exposure to sunlight.
  - ➢ **Zinc:** Found in lean meats, nuts, seeds, and legumes.

❖ **Antioxidant-Rich Foods:**
  - ➤ **Berries:** Antioxidants abound in strawberries, raspberries, and blueberries.
  - ➤ **Dark Leafy Greens:** Spinach, kale, and broccoli contain vitamins and antioxidants.
  - ➤ **Nuts and Seeds:** Almonds, sunflower seeds, and flaxseeds provide a dose of antioxidants.

Probiotics

  - ➤ Yoghurt with live cultures: Supports gut health and boosts the immune system.
  - ➤ Fermented Foods: Include kimchi, sauerkraut, and miso for a natural source of probiotics.
  - ➤ Kefir: A milk beverage that has fermented and contains healthy bacteria

❖ **Healthy Fats:**
  - ➤ **Avocados:** Avocados are high in vitamin E and monounsaturated fats.

- ➤ **Olive Oil:** Contains antioxidants and anti-inflammatory properties.
- ➤ **Fatty Fish:** Omega-3 fatty acids are found in salmon, mackerel, and trout.

❖ **Lean Proteins:**
- ➤ **Poultry:** Lean protein can be found in abundance in chicken and turkey.
- ➤ **Plant-based Proteins:** Beans, lentils, and tofu offer protein with additional nutrients.
- ➤ **Eggs:** Provide a complete protein source along with various nutrients.

❖ **Whole Grains:**
- ➤ **Quinoa, Brown Rice, Oats:** Whofibreains supply fibre, vitamins, and minerals.
- ➤ **Whole Wheat:** Choose whole wheat bread and pasta for added nutrients.

❖ **Colourful Vegetables:**
> ➤ **Carrots and sweet Potato are Peppers:** Packed with vitamins and antioxidants.
> ➤ **Cruciferous Vegetables:** Such as broccoli, cauliflower, and Brussels sprouts, are beneficial to overall health.

❖ **Hydration with Water and Herbal Teas:**
> ➤ Immune system performance and general health depend on maintaining adequate hydration.
> ➤ Herbal teas like chamomile and green tea offer antioxidants.

→ Remember, a diverse and balanced diet that incorporates these nutrient-rich foods contributes not only to immune health but also to overall vitality and longevity. Consistency in maintaining healthy eating habits forms a foundation for a resilient immune system.

CHAPTER THREE

HYDRATION AND IMMUNE HEALTH

Proper hydration is fundamental to maintaining overall health, and its impact extends to the immune system. Water plays a crucial role in supporting immune function and various physiological processes that contribute to the body's defence against infections. In this exploration of hydration and immune health, we'll delve into the significance of staying well-hydrated for a robust immune system.

❖ **Cellular Function and Immune Response:**
  - All cells, including immune cells, require water to function properly.
  - Adequate hydration helps transport nutrients to cells and remove waste products, facilitating efficient immune responses.

❖ **Lymphatic System Support:**
> ➢ The lymphatic system, a key
> component of the immune
> system, relies on proper
> hydration.
> ➢ Lymph, a fluid in the lymphatic
> system, transports immune cells
> and helps eliminate toxins from
> the body.

❖ **Mucosal Immunity:**
> ➢ Hydration is crucial for
> maintaining the integrity of
> mucous membranes in the
> respiratory and gastrointestinal
> tracts.
> ➢ Well-hydrated mucosal surfaces
> act as a barrier, preventing
> pathogens from entering the
> body.

❖ **Temperature Regulation:**
> ➢ Water helps regulate body
> temperature through sweating
> and evaporation.

> Maintaining a stable body temperature supports overall immune function.

❖ **Electrolyte Balance:**
> Proper hydration ensures a balance of electrolytes like sodium, potassium, and magnesium.
> Electrolytes are essential for nerve function, muscle contractions, and maintaining fluid balance, all of which impact immune health.

❖ **Hydration Tips for Immune Support:**
> **Drink Plenty of Water:** Aim for at least 8 glasses (64 ounces) of water daily, adjusting based on factors like age, weight, and physical activity.
> **Incorporate Hydrating Foods:** Fruits and vegetables with high water content, such as

watermelon, cucumber, and
oranges, contribute to overall
hydration.
➤ **Limit Dehydrating Substances:**
Reduce the intake of dehydrating
beverages like caffeinated and
alcoholic drinks.

❖ **Signs of Dehydration and
Immune Suppression:**
➤ Fatigue, dizziness, and
headaches can be signs of
dehydration.
➤ Prolonged dehydration may
compromise the immune system,
making the body more
susceptible to infections.

→ In the intricate web of factors influencing
immune health, hydration stands out as
a simple yet crucial component. By
prioritizing adequate water intake, you
not only support cellular function and
immune responses but also contribute
to the overall well-being of your body.

Stay mindful of your hydration levels, especially during times of increased physical activity, illness, or exposure to extreme temperatures, to ensure your immune system operates at its optimal capacity.

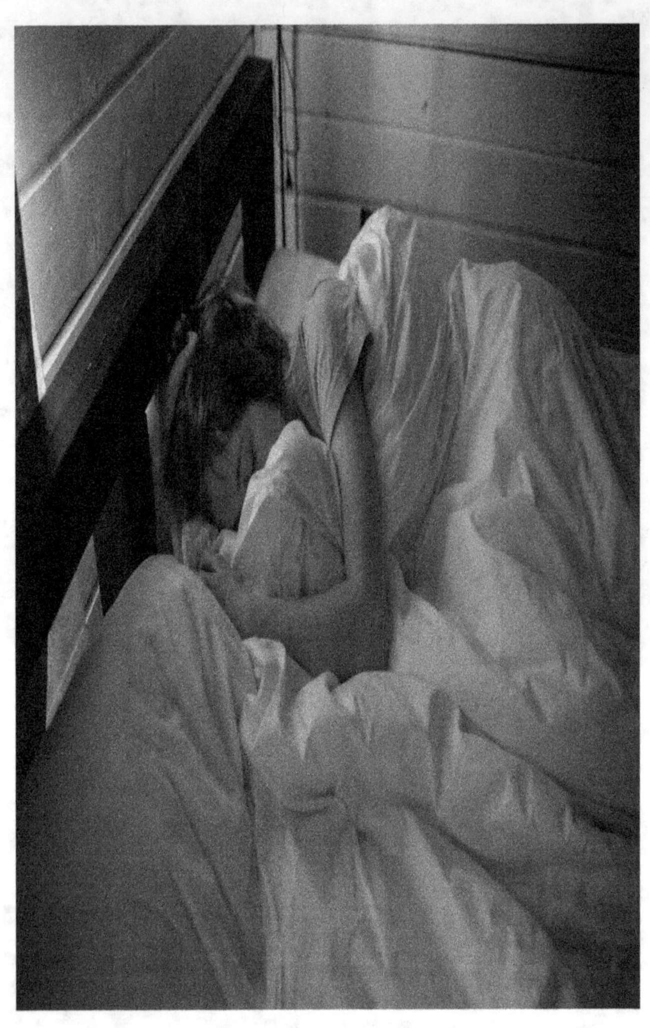

CHAPTER FOUR

ADEQUATE SLEEP FOR A STRONG IMMUNE SYSTEM

Sleep is often referred to as the body's natural healer, and its impact on overall health extends to the immune system. Adequate, quality sleep is essential for maintaining a robust defence against infections and illnesses. In this exploration of the connection between sleep and immune health, we'll delve into the importance of a good night's sleep for a resilient immune system.

- ❖ **The Immune System's Night Shift:**
    - ➢ During sleep, the body undergoes essential repair and restoration processes.
    - ➢ The immune system is particularly active, producing and releasing cytokines, antibodies, and immune cells that combat infections and inflammation.

* **Quality Sleep and Immune Cell Function:**
  - T cells, a type of immune cell, play a crucial role in identifying and destroying infected cells.
  - Adequate sleep enhances the function of T cells, promoting a more effective immune response.

* **Sleep Duration Matters:**
  - Consistent, sufficient sleep is key to maintaining a strong immune system.
  - Aim for 7-9 hours of sleep per night to optimize immune function and overall health.

* **Circadian Rhythm Regulation:**
  - Quality sleep helps regulate the body's circadian rhythm, the internal clock that influences various physiological processes.

> ➢ A well-regulated circadian rhythm ensures optimal timing for immune system activity.

❖ **Impact on Vaccination Response:**

> ➢ Studies suggest that well-rested individuals tend to generate a more robust immune response to vaccines.
> ➢ Adequate sleep can enhance the effectiveness of vaccinations.

❖ **Stress Reduction and Immune Support:**

> ➢ Quality sleep contributes to stress reduction, and chronic stress can suppress the immune system.
> ➢ Prioritizing restful sleep helps the body manage stress more effectively, supporting overall immune health.

- ❖ **Establishing Healthy Sleep Habits:**
    - ➢ Ensure a regular sleep routine by following the same bedtime and wake-up times every day, including on the weekends.
    - ➢ Establish a calming nighttime routine to let your body know when it's time to unwind.
    - ➢ Ensure a comfortable sleep environment, with a cool, dark, and quiet room.

- ❖ **Limiting Sleep Disruptors:**
    - ➢ Reduce the consumption of caffeine and electronic devices close to bedtime.
    - ➢ Manage stress through techniques such as meditation, deep breathing, or gentle exercises like yoga.
    - → In the hustle and bustle of daily life, it's easy to underestimate the profound impact that sleep has on our immune system. By recognizing the vital role of quality sleep in immune function and adopting healthy sleep habits, you

empower your body to better defend itself against pathogens and maintain optimal well-being. Prioritize your sleep, and you'll be investing in a stronger, more resilient immune system.

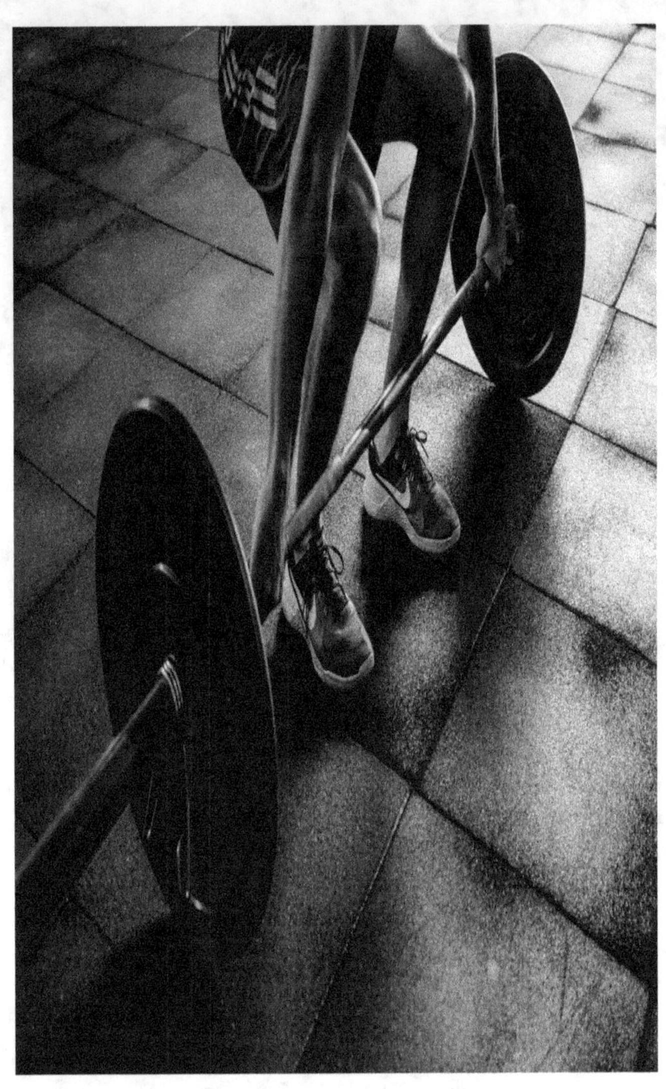

CHAPTER FIVE

REGULAR EXERCISE AND ITS IMPACT ON IMMUNITY

Regular exercise is a cornerstone of a healthy lifestyle, and its benefits extend beyond physical fitness to include a positive impact on the immune system. Engaging in consistent, moderate-intensity physical activity has been shown to enhance immune function and reduce the risk of infections. In this exploration of the relationship between exercise and immunity, we'll uncover the various ways in which staying active contributes to a stronger and more resilient immune system.

- ❖ **Immune Cell Activation:**
  - ➢ Exercise stimulates the circulation of immune cells, making them more efficient in patrolling the body and identifying potential threats.
  - ➢ Increased circulation allows immune cells to detect and respond to infections more rapidly.

❖ **Anti-Inflammatory Effects:**
  ➢ Chronic inflammation is linked to various diseases, including those affecting the immune system.
  ➢ Regular exercise helps regulate inflammation by promoting the production of anti-inflammatory cytokines.

❖ **Improved Blood Flow:**
  ➢ Enhanced blood circulation during exercise ensures that immune cells, antibodies, and nutrients are efficiently transported throughout the body.
  ➢ This increased circulation contributes to the optimal functioning of the immune system.

❖ **Stress Reduction:**
  ➢ Physical activity is a natural stress reliever, and chronic stress

can negatively impact immune
function.
> Regular exercise helps manage
stress levels, promoting a more
balanced and responsive immune
system.

❖ **Enhanced Vaccine Response:**
> Studies suggest that individuals
who engage in regular exercise
tend to exhibit a more robust
response to vaccinations.
> Exercise may contribute to the
improved effectiveness of
immunizations.

❖ **Promotion of Healthy Sleep:**
> Improved sleep quality is linked
to regular physical activity.
> Adequate, quality sleep is crucial
for a well-functioning immune
system.

❖ **Balancing Hormones:**
- ➤ Exercise helps regulate hormones such as cortisol and adrenaline, which play a role in immune function.
- ➤ Balanced hormone levels contribute to a healthier immune response.

❖ **Choosing the Right Exercise Routine:**
- ➤ Make time for moderate-intensity activities like cycling, swimming, or brisk walking for at least 150 minutes per week.
- ➤ Include strength training exercises to enhance muscle mass and overall fitness.
- ➤ Listen to your body and avoid overtraining, as excessive exercise can have the opposite effect on the immune system.

→ Incorporating regular exercise into your lifestyle is a proactive way to bolster your immune defences. Whether you prefer a brisk walk, a yoga session, or a weightlifting routine, staying active contributes to a well-rounded approach to immune health. By making physical activity a consistent part of your routine, you empower your body to better defend itself against infections and enjoy the numerous benefits of a stronger, more resilient immune system.

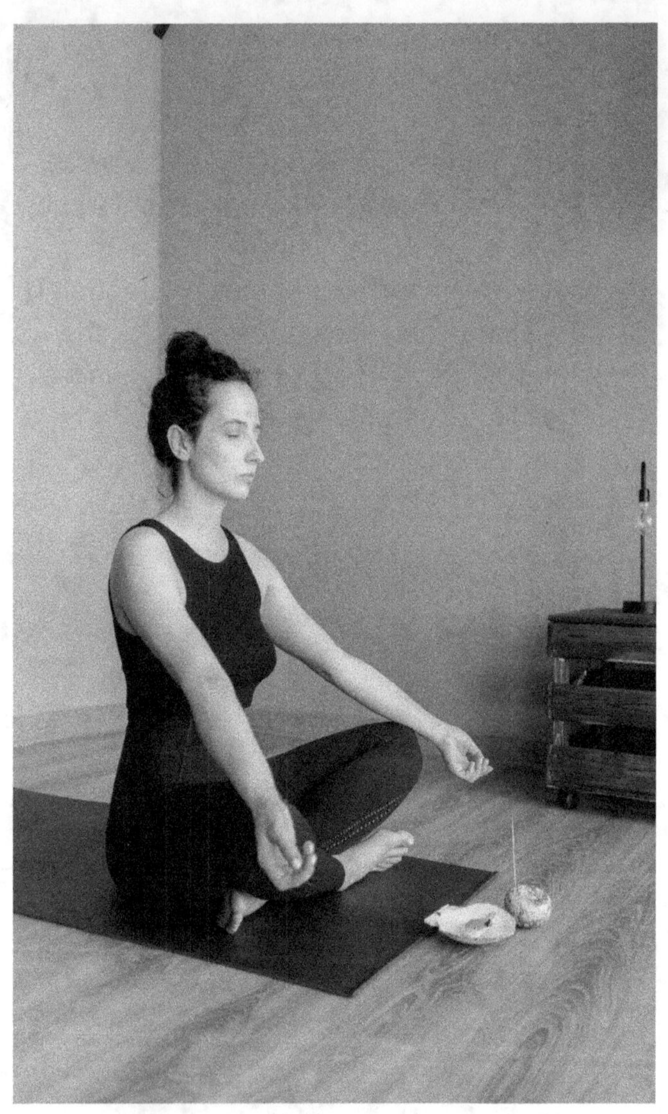

CHAPTER SIX

EFFECTIVE STRESS MANAGEMENT TECHNIQUES

In our fast-paced and demanding lives, stress has become a ubiquitous companion. However, managing stress is crucial for maintaining mental and physical well-being. Incorporating effective stress management techniques into your routine can enhance resilience, improve overall health, and foster a sense of balance. Let's explore a variety of techniques to help you navigate the challenges of daily life with greater ease.

- ❖ **Mindfulness Meditation:**
  - ➤ Through judgment-free present-moment attention, mindfulness meditation is practised.
  - ➤ Practices like deep breathing, body scans, and guided meditation can help reduce stress and promote a sense of calm.

- ❖ **Deep Breathing Exercises:**
    - ➢ Techniques such as diaphragmatic breathing or "belly breathing" can activate the body's relaxation response.
    - ➢ Inhale deeply through your nose, allowing your diaphragm to expand, and exhale slowly through your mouth.

- ❖ **Progressive Muscle Relaxation (PMR):**
    - ➢ PMR involves tensing and then gradually releasing different muscle groups, promoting physical and mental relaxation.
    - ➢ Consciously release tension by starting with your toes and working your way up to your head.

- ❖ **Yoga and Tai Chi:**
    - ➢ Both yoga and tai chi combine gentle movements with deep breathing and mindfulness.

➢ Regular practice can improve flexibility, reduce stress, and enhance overall well-being.

❖ **Exercise and Physical Activity:**
➢ Endorphins are the body's natural mood enhancers that are released when you exercise regularly.
➢ Find an activity you enjoy, whether it's walking, running, dancing, or cycling, and make it a consistent part of your routine.

❖ **Journaling:**
➢ Expressive writing allows you to release pent-up emotions and gain insights into your thoughts and feelings.
➢ Set aside time each day to write about your experiences, worries, and positive aspects of your life.

- ❖ **Social Connection:**
  - ➢ Sharing your thoughts and feelings with trusted friends or family members can provide emotional support.
  - ➢ Maintain meaningful connections and seek support when needed.

- ❖ **Time Management:**
  - ➢ Prioritize tasks and break them into smaller, manageable steps.
  - ➢ Set realistic goals and deadlines to avoid feeling overwhelmed.

- ❖ **Positive Affirmations:**
  - ➢ Replace negative thoughts with positive affirmations.
  - ➢ Repeat phrases that reinforce your strengths and ability to overcome challenges.

- ❖ **Hobbies and Leisure Activities:**
  - ➤ Take up anything you enjoy doing, be it gardening, reading, drawing, or listening to music.
  - ➤ Taking time for hobbies can provide a welcome break from stressors.

→ Incorporating stress management techniques into your daily life is a proactive investment in your well-being. Experiment with different approaches to discover what works best for you, and consider combining multiple techniques for a holistic approach. By prioritizing stress management, you empower yourself to navigate life's challenges with resilience, maintaining a sense of balance and mental clarity.

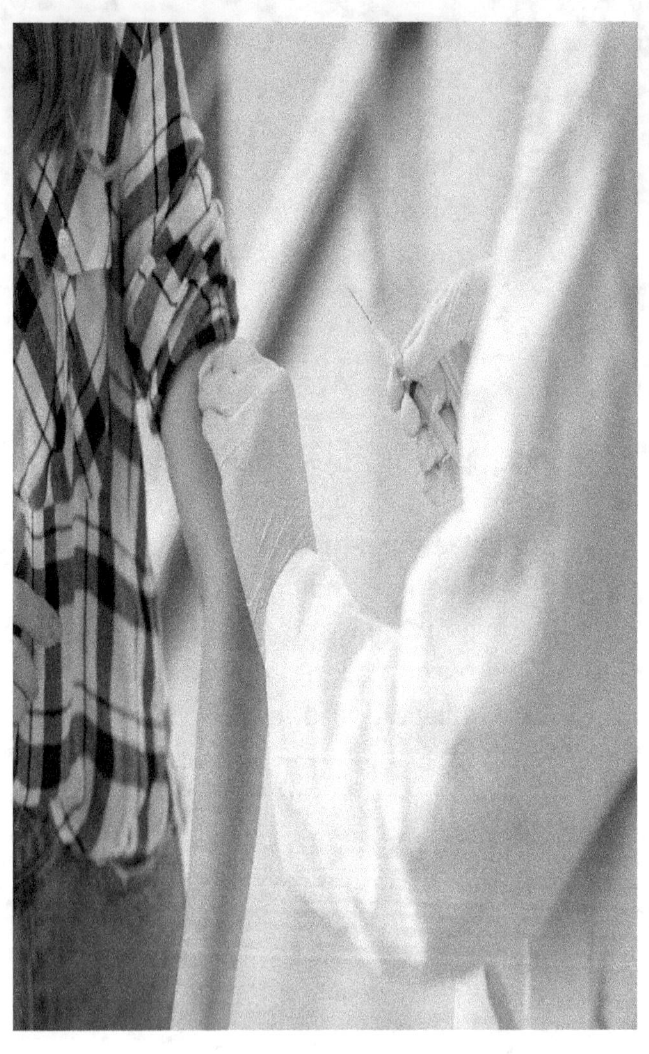

CHAPTER SEVEN

THE CRITICAL IMPORTANCE OF VACCINATIONS

Vaccinations are a cornerstone of public health, offering a powerful shield against a variety of infectious diseases. Their significance extends beyond individual protection to creating community-wide immunity, reducing the spread of diseases, and preventing outbreaks. In this exploration of the importance of vaccinations, we'll delve into the numerous benefits they provide to individuals, communities, and global health.

- ❖ **Disease Prevention:**
  - ➢ Vaccinations are designed to stimulate the immune system to recognize and combat specific pathogens, such as viruses or bacteria.
  - ➢ By preventing infections, vaccines play a pivotal role in reducing the incidence of diseases that can lead to severe illness, complications, and even death.

Community Immunity (Herd Immunity):

> Vaccinations contribute to community immunity, a phenomenon where a significant portion of the population is immune to a disease.
> When a high percentage of individuals are vaccinated, it helps protect those who cannot be vaccinated, such as infants, elderly individuals, or individuals with certain medical conditions.

❖ **Eradication of Diseases:**
> Vaccination campaigns have successfully led to the eradication of some diseases, such as smallpox.
> Continued efforts aim to eliminate other diseases, like polio and measles, through widespread vaccination initiatives.

- ❖ **Reduction of Disease Spread:**
  - ➢ Vaccinated individuals are less likely to contract and spread diseases to others.
  - ➢ This "break in the chain of transmission" helps control the spread of infectious agents within communities.

- ❖ **Protection of Vulnerable Populations:**
  - ➢ Certain populations, such as newborns, pregnant women, and individuals with weakened immune systems, are more susceptible to severe complications from vaccine-preventable diseases.
  - ➢ Vaccinations offer a layer of protection for these vulnerable groups.

- ❖ **Economic and Social Impact:**
  - ➢ Vaccinations contribute to economic stability by preventing

the economic burden associated
with treating and controlling
infectious diseases.
➢ Healthy populations are more
productive, leading to stronger
and more resilient societies.

❖ **Global Health Security:**
➢ In an interconnected world,
vaccinations play a crucial role in
global health security.
➢ Preventing the spread of
infectious diseases across
borders helps protect populations
worldwide.

❖ **Advancements in Research and
Technology:**
➢ Ongoing research and
technological advancements in
vaccine development contribute
to the creation of more effective
and targeted vaccines.

> ➢ Continued innovation helps
address emerging threats and
evolving pathogens.

→ Vaccinations are a cornerstone of public
health, offering a proven and effective
means of preventing the spread of
infectious diseases. By ensuring
widespread vaccine coverage,
individuals and communities can
collectively contribute to the well-being
of society, protect vulnerable
populations, and work towards the goal
of global health security. The importance
of vaccinations cannot be overstated, as
they represent a powerful tool in our
collective efforts to safeguard health and
build a resilient and thriving global
community.

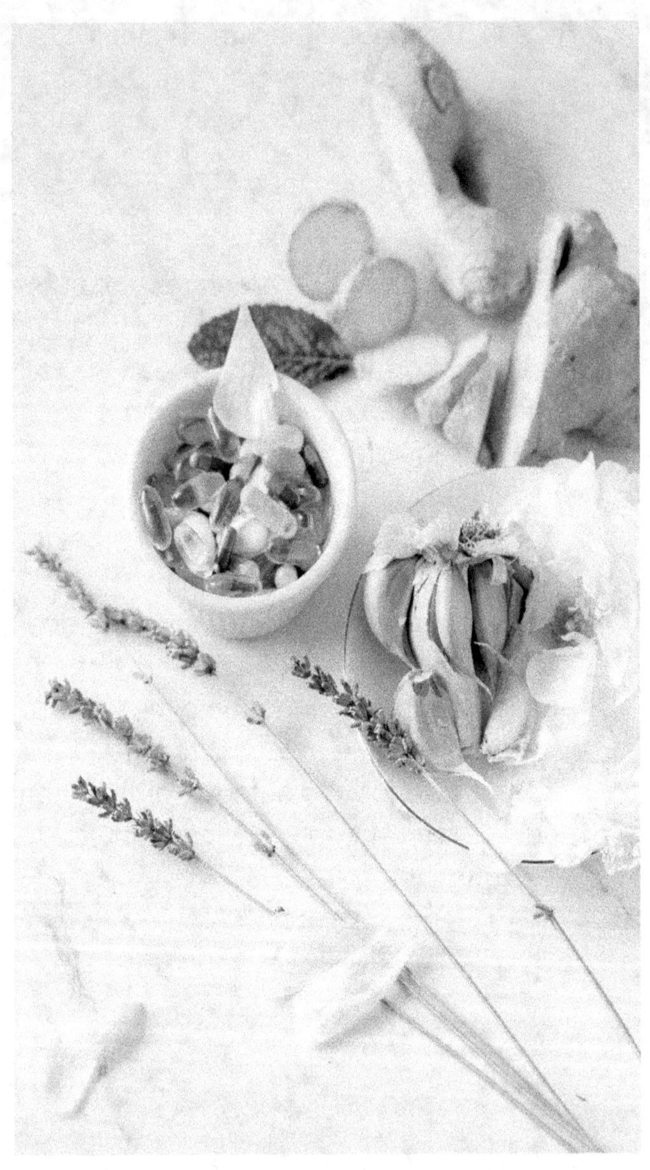

CHAPTER EIGHT

HERBAL SUPPLEMENTS FOR IMMUNE SUPPORT

Since ancient times, herbal supplements have been utilized as all-natural treatments to promote health and well-being. In recent years, there has been a growing interest in the potential of certain herbs to enhance immune function. While herbal supplements are not a substitute for a healthy lifestyle and medical guidance, they can play a complementary role in supporting the immune system. In this exploration of herbal supplements for immune support, we'll delve into some notable herbs and their potential benefits.

❖ **Echinacea:**
- ➢ **Benefits:** Known for its immune-boosting properties, echinacea is believed to stimulate the immune system and reduce the severity and duration of colds.
- ➢ **Usage:** Typically taken as a supplement or in herbal teas.

❖ **Garlic:**
  - ➢ ***Benefits:*** Garlic possesses antimicrobial and immune-enhancing properties. It may help the immune system combat infections and reduce the risk of getting sick.
  - ➢ ***Usage:*** Fresh garlic in meals or as a supplement.

❖ **Ginger:**
  - ➢ ***Benefits:*** Ginger has anti-inflammatory and antioxidant properties. It might assist in lowering inflammation and adjusting the immunological response.
  - ➢ ***Usage:*** Commonly consumed as fresh ginger in foods or as ginger tea.

❖ **Turmeric:**
  - ➢ ***Benefits:*** Curcumin, the active compound in turmeric, has potent anti-inflammatory and antioxidant

effects, which may support the immune system.

> *Usage:* Often taken as a supplement or incorporated into curries and beverages.

❖ **Astragalus:**

> **Benefits:** Used in traditional Chinese medicine, astragalus is believed to support the immune system by stimulating the production of white blood cells.
> **Usage:** Typically taken as a supplement or in herbal teas.

❖ **Reishi Mushroom:**

> **Benefits:** Reishi mushrooms have been associated with immune-modulating effects. They may help regulate the immune response and improve overall immune function.
> **Usage:** Available in supplement form or as an ingredient in some teas.

❖ **Elderberry:**

> ➤ ***Benefits:*** Elderberry is rich in antioxidants and may help reduce the severity and duration of cold and flu symptoms.
> ➤ ***Usage:*** Often consumed as elderberry syrup, capsules, or in herbal teas.

❖ **Licorice Root:**

> ➤ ***Benefits:*** Licorice root has anti-inflammatory and immune-modulating properties. The respiratory system may benefit from its support.
> ➤ ***Usage:*** Available in supplement form or as a tea.

❖ **Holy Basil (Tulsi):**

> ➤ ***Benefits:*** Holy Basil is revered in Ayurvedic medicine for its adaptogenic properties. It may

help the body adapt to stress and support immune function.
> *Usage:* Consumed as a tea or supplement.

❖ **Green Tea:**
> *Benefits:* Rich in polyphenols, green tea has antioxidant and anti-inflammatory properties that may contribute to overall immune health.
> *Usage:* Consumed as a beverage or as a supplement.

→ While herbal supplements can be valuable additions to a holistic approach to immune support, it's crucial to consult with healthcare professionals before incorporating them into your routine. These supplements should complement, not replace, a healthy diet, regular exercise, and other evidence-based measures for maintaining overall well-being. By integrating carefully selected herbal supplements, individuals

may harness the potential benefits of
nature to reinforce their immune
defences and support a healthier, more
resilient lifestyle.

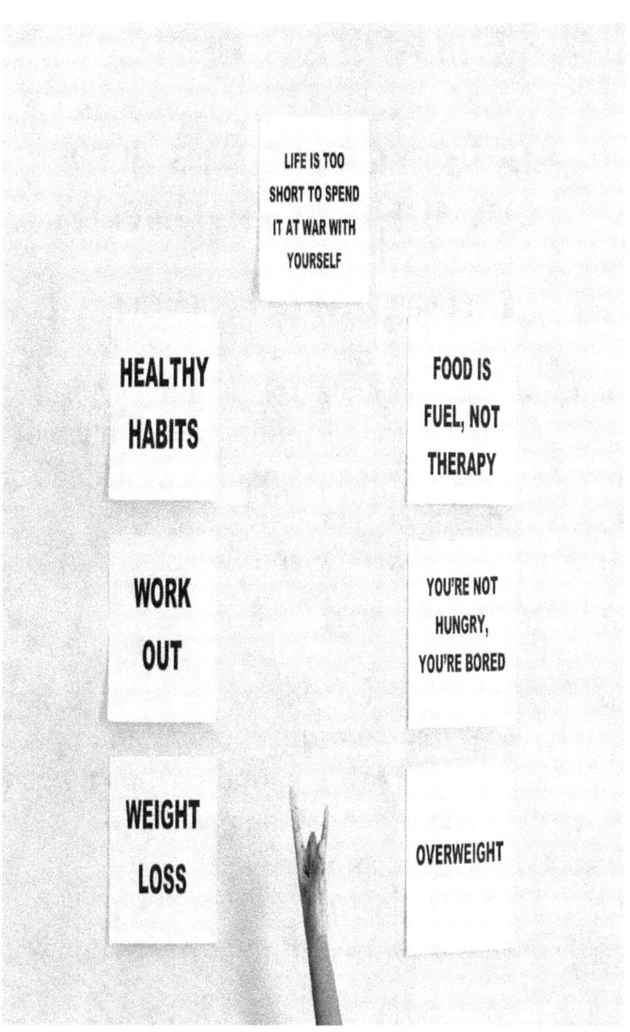

LIFE IS TOO SHORT TO SPEND IT AT WAR WITH YOURSELF
HEALTHY HABITS
FOOD IS FUEL, NOT THERAPY
WORK OUT
YOU'RE NOT HUNGRY, YOU'RE BORED
WEIGHT LOSS
OVERWEIGHT

CHAPTER NINE

LIFESTYLE HABITS FOR IMMUNE BOOSTING

A robust immune system is essential for safeguarding our health, and certain lifestyle habits can play a pivotal role in fortifying our body's natural defences. In this exploration of immune-boosting lifestyle habits, we'll focus on three key practices: Hand hygiene, Sun exposure for Vitamin D, and Social connections.

- ❖ **Hand Hygiene:**
    - ➤ *Importance:* Proper hand hygiene is a fundamental practice to prevent the spread of infections.
    - ➤ *Habit Tips:*
        - Wash hands regularly with soap and water for at least 20 seconds, especially after being in public places or touching surfaces.
        - In the absence of soap and water, use hand

sanitizer that has at least
60% alcohol.
- Keep your hands clean
  while handling your face,
  especially your lips, nose,
  and eyes.

❖ **Sun Exposure for Vitamin D:**
  - ➤ ***Importance:*** Vitamin D plays a
    crucial role in immune function,
    and sunlight is a natural source.
  - ➤ ***Habit Tips:***
    - Spend time outdoors,
      aiming for about 10-30
      minutes of sun exposure
      on arms, face, and legs
      several times a week.
    - Be mindful of sunscreen
      use; while important for
      skin health, it can reduce
      Vitamin D synthesis.
    - Include Vitamin D-rich
      foods in your diet, such as
      fatty fish, fortified dairy
      products, and mushrooms.

- ❖ **Social Connections:**
  - ➤ *Importance:* Emotional well-being and social connections have a direct impact on immune health.
  - ➤ *Habit Tips:*
    - ■ Cultivate and maintain positive relationships with friends, family, and community.
    - ■ Engage in regular social activities, whether in person or virtually, to foster a sense of connection.
    - ■ Practice active listening and open communication to strengthen interpersonal bonds.

- ❖ **Balanced Nutrition:**
  - ➤ *Importance:* A well-balanced diet provides essential nutrients that support immune function.
  - ➤ *Habit Tips:*
    - ■ Eat a diet rich in whole grains, lean meats, fruits, veggies, and healthy fats.

- Prioritize foods rich in vitamins and minerals, such as Vitamin C, Vitamin D, zinc, and antioxidants.
- Limit the intake of processed foods, excessive sugar, and unhealthy fats.

❖ Adequate Sleep:

➢ **Importance:** Quality sleep is crucial for immune system function and overall health.

➢ **Habit Tips:**

- Set a regular sleep routine with a goal of seven to nine hours each night.
- To tell your body when it's time to wind down, establish a calming sleep routine.
- Ensure a comfortable sleep environment, with a cool, dark room and minimal electronic device use before bedtime.

❖ **Regular Physical Activity:**
> ➤ *Importance:* Exercise contributes to overall health and can enhance immune function.
> ➤ *Habit Tips:*
>> ■ Make time for moderate-intense exercise every week—at least 150 minutes of it.
>> ■ Incorporate a variety of cardiovascular, strength, and flexibility workouts into your training regimen.
>> ■ To include fitness into your routine on a long-term basis, find things you enjoy doing.

➔ Incorporating these immune-boosting lifestyle habits into your daily routine can contribute to a resilient defence against infections and promote overall well-being. By cultivating good hand hygiene, embracing sunlight for Vitamin D, fostering social connections, maintaining a balanced diet, prioritizing sleep, and engaging in regular physical activity, you empower your body to function optimally and build a foundation for a healthy and vibrant life.

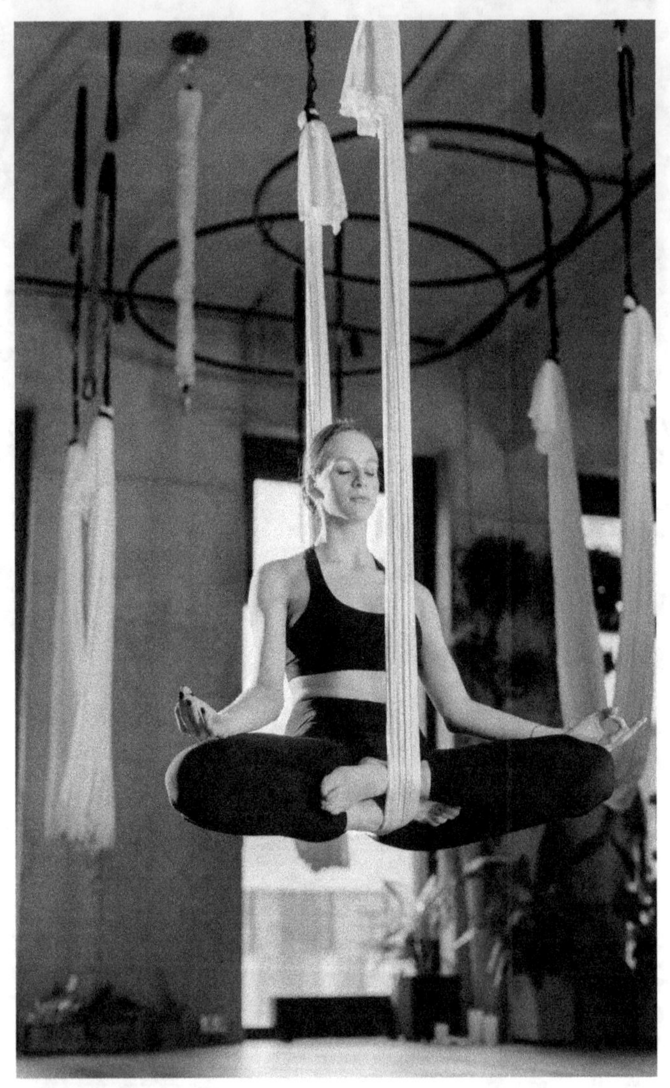

CHAPTER TEN

BALANCING IMMUNE-BOOSTING PRACTICES FOR OPTIMAL HEALTH

Building a resilient immune system involves incorporating a variety of healthy habits into your daily routine. While individual practices contribute to immune support, it's essential to strike a balance to avoid extremes that may lead to unintended consequences. In this exploration of balancing immune-boosting practices, we'll delve into key considerations for achieving optimal health.

- ❖ **Diverse Nutrient Intake:**
  - ➢ ***Balancing Act:*** While it's crucial to include immune-boosting nutrients in your diet, focusing on a single nutrient excessively may not be beneficial.
  - ➢ ***Tip:*** Embrace a colourful and diverse diet, including a variety of fruits, vegetables, whole grains, lean proteins, and healthy fats.

❖ **Sun Exposure and Sunscreen Use:**
  - ➤ ***Balancing Act:*** Sun exposure is vital for Vitamin D synthesis, but excessive sun exposure without protection can lead to skin damage.
  - ➤ ***Tip:*** Aim for moderate sun exposure while being mindful of sunscreen use, especially during extended periods outdoors.

❖ **Hand Hygiene vs. Microbial Exposure:**
  - ➤ ***Balancing Act:*** Overzealous hand hygiene may compromise the natural development of immune tolerance.
  - ➤ ***Tip:*** Practice regular hand hygiene, especially in high-risk situations, but allow for reasonable exposure to everyday microbes to support immune system education.

- ❖ **Social Connections and Personal Space:**
    - ➢ *Balancing Act:* While social connections are essential, finding a balance with personal space is crucial to prevent the spread of infections.
    - ➢ *Tip:* Foster social connections while respecting personal boundaries, and be mindful of physical distancing during contagious periods.

- ❖ **Exercise Intensity:**
    - ➢ *Balancing Act:* Intense exercise can enhance immune function, but excessive or exhaustive training may lead to immune suppression.
    - ➢ *Tip:* Incorporate a mix of moderate-intensity and high-intensity exercises into your routine, allowing for sufficient rest and recovery.

❖ **Sleep Quantity and Quality:**

> *Balancing Act:* Both insufficient and excessive sleep can have negative effects on immune health.

> *Tip:* Aim for 7-9 hours of quality sleep per night, maintaining a consistent sleep schedule and creating a conducive sleep environment.

❖ **Stress Management Techniques:**

> *Balancing Act:* Chronic stress can compromise the immune system, but a stress-free life is often unrealistic.

> *Tip:* Adopt stress management techniques such as meditation, deep breathing, or yoga to strike a balance and build resilience.

- ❖ **Vaccination and Natural Immunity:**
  - ➢ *Balancing Act:* Relying solely on natural immunity may leave you susceptible to preventable diseases, while vaccines provide targeted protection.
  - ➢ *Tip:* Embrace vaccination as a proactive measure while acknowledging the importance of natural immune responses.

→ Achieving a balance in immune-boosting practices is key to fostering optimal health. Rather than focusing exclusively on one aspect, aim for a holistic approach that incorporates a variety of habits. By striking harmony in your diet, sun exposure, hygiene practices, social interactions, exercise routine, sleep patterns, stress management, and vaccination decisions, you create a comprehensive foundation for a resilient immune system and overall well-being. For individualized advice catered to your particular health needs, always seek the advice of medical professionals.

CHAPTER ELEVEN

CONCLUSION

In the pursuit of optimal health and a resilient immune system, it's clear that a multifaceted approach is the key to success. By incorporating a variety of immune-boosting practices into your lifestyle, you create a synergistic effect that supports your body's natural defences. From maintaining a balanced diet, embracing sunlight for Vitamin D, and practising good hygiene, to fostering social connections, getting adequate sleep, and managing stress, each element contributes to the overall tapestry of well-being.

Striking a balance among these practices is paramount. While individual efforts are crucial, an excessive focus on one aspect may lead to unintended consequences. The goal is not perfection but rather a holistic and sustainable integration of healthy habits into your daily life.

It's important to recognize that health is a dynamic and individualized journey. Factors such as age, underlying health conditions, and lifestyle choices all play a role. Consulting with healthcare professionals for personalized guidance ensures that your approach aligns with your unique needs.

As we navigate the complexities of modern life, the importance of a well-rounded immune-boosting strategy cannot be overstated. By making informed choices, fostering resilience, and embracing a comprehensive view of health, you empower yourself to live vibrantly and proactively contribute to the well-being of those around you.

Remember, the path to a strong immune system is a journey, not a destination. By maintaining a commitment to balanced, evidence-based practices, you embark on a lifelong quest for optimal health and a resilient immune system